I0435732

Disclaimer: The contents of this book may not be construed as a medical diagnosis, treatment, advice, claim, or substitute for a physician's care. Consult a physician or other health care provider before starting a weight loss or exercise program. Dr. Susan Williamson's results are not typical, and she cannot guarantee you will have the same results. Your results depend on many factors such as your current state of health, age, metabolism, hormone balance, lifestyle, activity level, etc. It should not be used in place of a visit, consultation with or the advice of a physician or other qualified health care provider. The authors and the publisher shall have neither liability nor responsibility to any person or entity with respect to any loss or damages arising from the information contained in this book.

The statements in this HCG Diet: Doctor's Guide Book have not been evaluated by the FDA. FDA Disclaimer: HCG is not FDA approved for weight loss. There is no substantial evidence that it increases weight loss beyond that resulting from caloric restriction, that it causes a more attractive or "normal" distribution of fat, or that it decreases the hunger and discomfort associated with calorie-restricted diets. The HCG diet is not recommended for those who currently have cancer or have had cancer in the past, as HCG is a hormone. It is always best to consult with your physician prior to starting any diet or weight loss plan even if you do not have any known or existing health conditions.

Table of Contents

About the Author:

Dr. Susan Williamson NMD

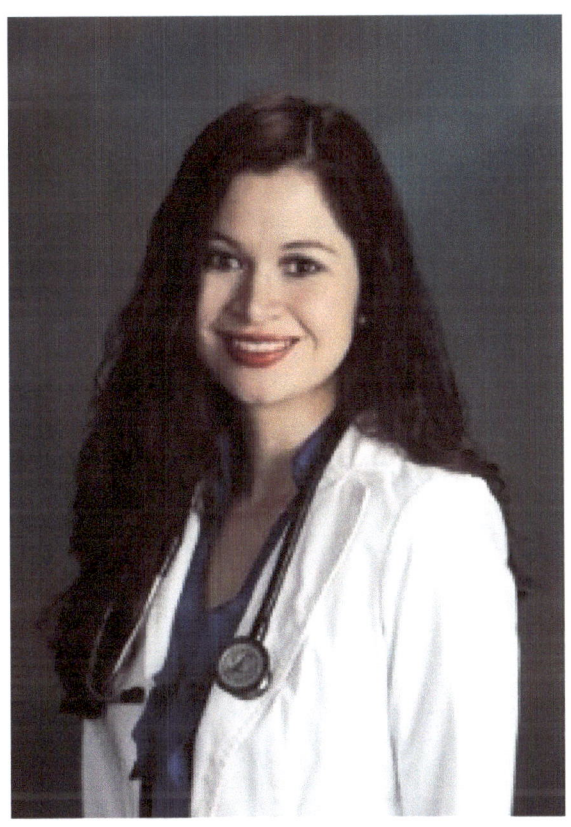

Dr. Susan Williamson received her Bachelor of Science Summa Cum Laude in Biological Sciences with a minor in Chemistry and Psychology from Youngstown State University in Youngstown, Ohio. Immediately after graduating from college, Dr. Williamson moved to Arizona from Pennsylvania to attend Southwest College of Naturopathic Medicine where she obtained her **Doctorate in Naturopathic Medicine**, **ranking first in her class and receiving the Highest Academic Achievement Award.** She is a **licensed Naturopathic Physician** in the state of Arizona and is the founder of **W Clinic of Integrative Medicine.** Dr. Williamson has advanced, post-graduate training in bio-identical hormone replacement with The American Academy of Anti-Aging Medicine. She is a member of the Arizona Naturopathic Medical Association (AzNMA). Dr. Williamson firmly believes in finding and treating the underlying cause of disease versus suppressing symptoms. She treats a wide variety of health conditions ranging from acute to chronic disease. She also specializes in the treatment of hormone imbalances, Anti-Aging Medicine, thyroid disorders, weight loss including using the HCG Diet in her practice, as well as utilizes clinical nutrition in her medical practice to treat disease. She enjoys spending time with her husband Josh, her son Joshua, and her dog, Snowy.

Dr. Williamson's HCG Diet Before and After Pictures

Dr. Williamson gained a total of 65 lbs during pregnancy. She lost 15 lbs after giving birth to her son but was left with 50 lbs to lose. 50 lbs of her total 65 lbs was lost using the HCG diet within 5 months with no exercise*.

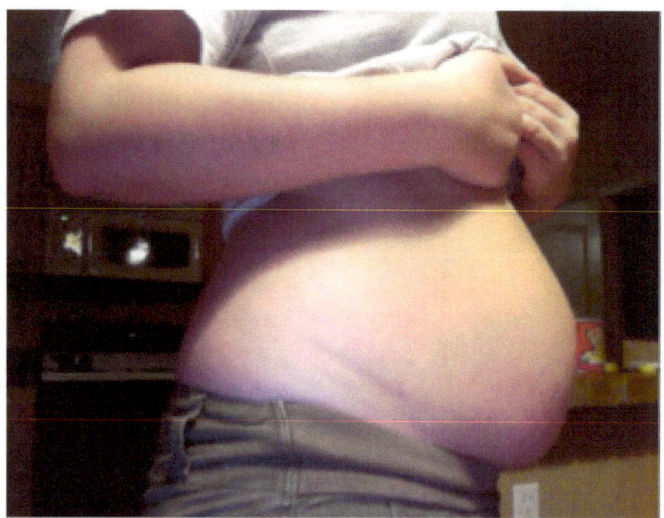

Before- After baby was born

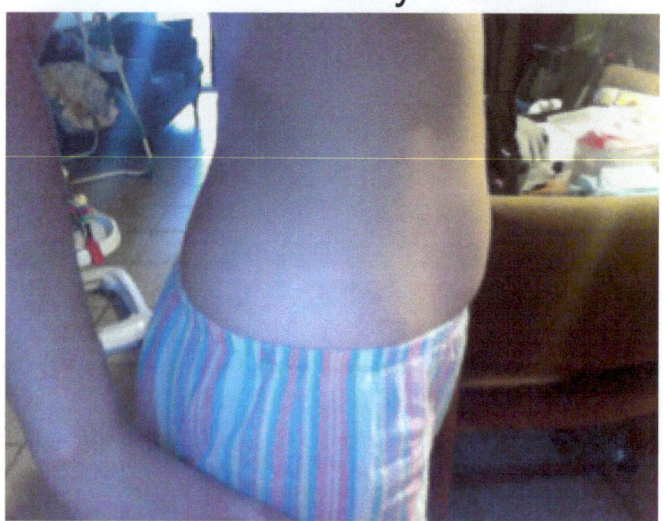

After HCG diet

*Individual results may vary. Weight loss depends on many factors such as metabolic rate, activity level, adherence to a diet, and exercise. It is recommended to undergo laboratory testing and a medical evaluation to determine if your metabolism and hormones are balanced prior to starting a weight loss program, and to determine if you are healthy enough for a weight loss program. FDA Disclaimer: HCG is not FDA approved for weight loss. There is no substantial evidence that it increases weight loss beyond that resulting from caloric restriction, that it causes a more attractive or "normal" distribution of fat, or that it decreases the hunger and discomfort associated with calorie-restricted diets. The HCG diet is not recommended for those who currently have cancer or have had cancer in the past, as HCG is a hormone. It is always best to consult with your physician prior to starting any diet or weight loss plan even if you do not have any existing health conditions.

History of HCG

During the 1950s, Dr. A.T.W. Simeons, an endocrinologist, discovered that low doses of HCG in obese patients allowed their body to mobilize and use "abnormal fat" stores as a source of energy, thus leading to considerable weight loss. He also found that HCG in pregnant women served as a protective mechanism for the fetus should the mother not consume an adequate amount of calories. Capitalizing on this knowledge, he found that combining HCG with a very low calorie diet (VLCD) produced dramatic weight loss at the rate of 1 to 3 pounds per day. It is speculated that In a person who is not taking HCG, this same VLCD would put the body in starvation mode and the opposite would occur—fat would be stored rather than being mobilized for energy. Dr. Simeons also speculated that HCG resets the body's "thermostat," the hypothalamus, which is the body's control station for metabolic rate, hunger, thirst, and body temperature which also contributes to the dramatic weight loss seen with the HCG diet.

How does HCG theoretically work?

One pound of fat is equal to 3,500 calories. Jogging for 1 mile burns about 100 calories. If you're 50 pounds overweight, you need to jog from San Francisco to Dallas (1,750 miles) to burn 50 pounds (mathematically that is, without taking different metabolism speeds into consideration). However, if it were that simple to lose weight then many more Americans would be jogging from coast to coast. Many Americans work out regularly and burn the calories but can't seem to lose the weight. The reason why? They are burning the wrong calories.

An Example of How HCG may work

If a person's normal metabolism requires 2000 calories per day, and that person is consuming only 500 calories per day on the HCG diet, then the remaining 1500 calories will come from "abnormal fat" stores (i.e. the stomach, hips, thighs, buttocks, back, under arms). These abnormal fat stores are often the stubborn areas that don't seem to diminish with regular dieting.

An Explanation: 3 types of fats are found within the human body according to Dr. Simeons:

- **Structural fat:** serves as a kind of "packing material" for the body; Structural fat fills in empty space between organs.

- **Normal Fat**: the fat that the body uses for energy when calorie intake is less than bodily demands.

- **Abnormal fat:** excessive and abnormal accumulations of fixed deposits of fat located throughout the body and associated with obesity. During nutritional emergencies (i.e. not having adequate amount of calories) the body is unable to use this fat for energy.

Dr. Simeons believed that when exercising or restricting food intake, the body relies on and consumes the normal fat reserves. The body cannot access the abnormal fat accumulations. Dr. Simeons speculated that the use of the HCG hormone releases abnormal fat deposits and makes the fat available for consumption by the body.

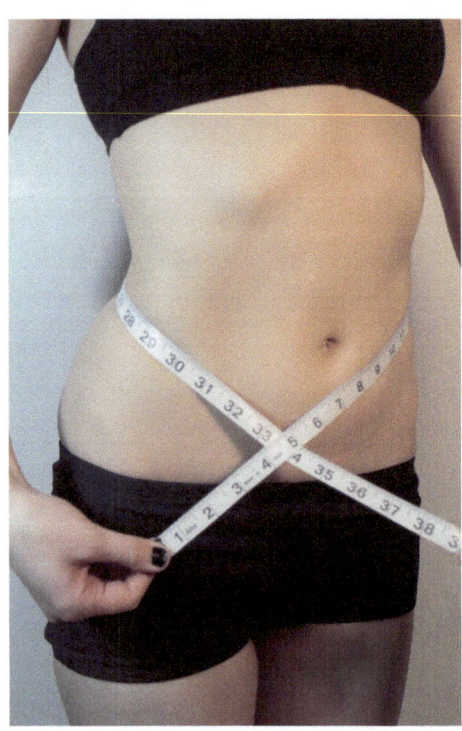

Before you start the HCG Diet: Tips and Tricks:

1. Make sure you are mentally prepared! This is number one on the list of things to do prior to starting the HCG diet. It is best to not do the diet near Holidays or special events such as Birthday parties or Weddings as this can set you up for self-sabotage or failure if your will power is not strong. Some people are able to make it through such events without "cheating" or eating off the diet, however I recommend not even having the temptation around to ensure success.

2. Plan your meals and purchase your foods ahead of time. It is much easier to do the diet when you know what your meal plan consists of and have the food on hand.

3. Purchase a food scale to measure the weight of your food and to manage portion sizes. I purchased a non-digital food scale for $5.00 at the store. You can however purchase a nice digital food scale but a simple one will also serve the purpose.

4. Remove junk foods/temptations in the house. You can eat your junk food prior to starting the HCG diet, throw it away, or eat it during the Loading Phase. But once you start the actual HCG diet itself, it is best to not even have these foods in your home. Out of sight, out of mind. Also during the "Loading Phase" one does not have to gorge him/herself into a food coma. When I did my loading phase I ate a hamburger and some frozen yogurt on day 1 of loading, and then indulged in some guacamole and wings the next day (day 2 of loading) and did not go overboard on the loading. I knew I did not want to gain any additional weight, which would have set me back. Some people will eat so much during loading days that they gain 3 lbs in those 2 days which they will then have to lose, causing them a little bit of a set back.

5. It is a great idea to track your foods on an online website or phone application such as My Fitness Pal®. I specifically used My Fitness Pal® to track my weight loss and to pre-plan my meals so that I could calculate out my exact amount of calories (AND CARBOHYDRATES). I

will discuss the importance of tracking carbohydrates later on in this book. This is something that is not discussed in the original Dr. Simeons protocol, but is important for rapid weight loss on the HCG diet.

6. Make sure you have HCG friendly beauty and health products for the diet. This will be discussed later in the book with specific product recommendations later in the book, something that is not discussed in the original Dr. Simeoons protocol.

7. It may be necessary to purchase in-between clothing sizes as you lose the weight if you do not have a wide array of clothing sizes in your closet. I recommend visiting your local thrift store as your clothing size will change rapidly during the diet and you may change clothing size in as little as a week at a time.

8. <u>It is best to have prescription HCG obtained from a physician for the diet.</u> Homeopathic preparations are commercially available, however being that it is homeopathic, it means that the preparation contains no measureable amount of HCG in the formulation and is thus only water. Homeopathic preparations do work, but when used in the right way. I use homeopathy in my medical practice and homeopathic HCG is not used in the way that homeopathy is used. Homeopathy is based off of the principal of like cures like. Hundreds of years ago people would take dilute amounts of substances and record the symptoms it caused them. When one takes a homeopathic remedy, they want to take a remedy that causes the same symptoms that were elicited during the proving and they want to take the remedy that best matches up with their symptoms. Taking a remedy that most closely matches up with their current symptoms results in those symptoms being "cancelled out" and thus the symptoms go away and the individual gets better. Homeopathic HCG is not even listed in the homeopathic pharmacopeia because it has never undergone a proving to see what symptoms it elicits in healthy people. So taking homeopathic HCG in this manner is incorrect and probably does not work. It's analogous to taking homeopathic opiates for pain relief, which is not how homeopathy works. So please make sure you are using prescription

grade HCG. Some people have been successful using the homeopathic HCG preparations however this was probably due to the placebo effect.

9. Hormones: *Make sure your hormones are balanced before you start the HCG diet or any weight loss program for that matter!* Hormones control all when it comes to weight loss and body composition. Thyroid controls your metabolism while estrogen, progesterone, and testosterone maintains your sexual organs, skin, hair, and lean muscle mass.

It is always a good idea to have your thyroid hormone levels checked prior to starting a weight loss program. The thyroid produces thyroid hormones, which controls your basal metabolic rate (i.e. how fast you burn calories at rest). An optimal Thyroid Stimulating Hormone (TSH) level is between a 0.3 to 2.0. Note I mentioned "optimal," not "normal." Recent studies have shown that the "normal" thyroid range is set too high resulting in people being misdiagnosed/not diagnosed with a hypothyroid when they should be. A slow metabolism will result in inability to lose weight, slow weight loss, and/or weight gain as well as other symptoms such as depression, fatigue, hair loss, dry skin, water retention, decreased libido, anxiety, slow reflexes, etc. You may have only one symptom if you do have a hypothyroid but please be sure to have this checked before starting a weight loss program.

If you are a peri-menopausal or post-menopausal woman, it is a good idea to have your female hormones estrogen, progesterone, and testosterone checked in addition to the thyroid. Low sex hormones will result in inability to lose weight, slow weight loss, and/or weight gain.

If you are a man, it is best to also have your testosterone and estrogen levels checked in addition to the thyroid prior to starting the weight loss program. I have seen young men as early as 20 years old in my practice who have low testosterone levels and/or high estrogen levels. Testosterone maintains your sex drive as well as your lean muscle mass. The more lean muscle mass one has, the faster the metabolic rate. If you are a male and your belly sticks out further than your chest, then chances are you are low in testosterone.

10. If you are a woman of childbearing age, make sure you are NOT PREGNANT. Please be sure to take a pregnancy test if your periods are irregular or if your last menstrual period is late/overdue.

11. If you are a woman of childbearing age, make sure to use contraception (such as condoms) as HCG can make you very fertile and can result in ovarian hyper-stimulation in which you ovulate more than one egg. HCG is also used as a fertility drug to stimulate ovulation in women for those who are dealing with infertility, and it is also used in men to boost testosterone production. I do not recommend using HCG while taking oral contraceptive pills. HCG Diet should also not be done if breastfeeding. However women on Bio-identical hormone replacement therapy should continue their medications as directed, even if they are using hormone creams. I have seen better weight loss results in menopausal women who continue their bio-identical hormones during the course of the HCG diet. The reason I do not recommend using HCG while on the oral contraceptive pill is because the HCG stimulates the ovaries while the birth control is trying to prevent ovulation (opposite effects). Also oral contraceptive pills contain 10 times higher dosages of hormones than do bio-identical hormones and are synthetic, not natural, which poses more risks for adverse interactions.

12. It is a good idea to get body measurements prior to starting the diet, and then once a week thereafter to monitor progress. Some people will see more inches come off than pounds. The best areas to measure are around the arms (but be sure to measure 4-6 inches above the elbow and record this) so that you are measuring around the same part of the upper arm each time. Also around the thigh (again measure 4-6 inches above the top of the knee cap and record this) so that you are measuring the same part of the upper thigh each time. And around the abdomen at the level of the umbilicus/belly button and around the hips.

13. Soy lecithin or Sunflower lecithin can be taken during the HCG protocol to aid your liver and gallbladder in the breakdown of fat. Due to the rapid weight loss on the diet, your liver and gallbladder become stressed as they have to process all of the fat you are dumping/circulating in your system. These supplements can be purchased over the counter.

The HCG Diet: Basic Rules

- **200 IU of HCG daily (*except during menstruation if you are a menstruating female*).** Some people will do ok on a lower dose, such as 150 IU, however I was finding that I had to adjust 50% or more of patients up to the full dose for satiety/appetite control which has led me to prescribe 200 IU for my HCG patients.
    - NOTE: If using ORAL HCG: If you are using oral, sublingual HCG, then you will need to take the 200 IU twice a day- AM and PM as the HCG does not stay in your system as long as when you do injections.
- For menstruating women, it is best to start the program immediately following menstruation since the injections will need to be stopped during menstruation. **Continuing the injections during menstruation may lead to excessively heavy bleeding and/or increased risk of pregnancy, or a developed immunity against the effects of the HCG. Therefore, NO INJECTIONS ARE PERMITTED *DURING MENSTRUATION*. Once the menstrual period stops, then HCG injections are resumed daily.**
- **NO EXERCISE IS ALLOWED WHILE ON THE 500 Calorie Diet (aka. The Reduction Phase)** (20 minutes of light walking per day is acceptable if you must have some physical activity).
- **NO ARTIFICIAL SWEETENERS ALLOWED.** Stevie, an all natural zero calorie sweetener derived from the stevia plant (Rebiana), may be used as a sweetener. Stevia comes in many flavors and now allows for many possibilities when it comes to flavoring food and drinks. Mixing stevia with mineral water makes a great "mock soda." NO DIET SODA! It is also recommended that if you are a Diet Soda drinker that you stop drinking it altogether as the artificial sweetener in the diet sodas are known to cause weight gain! One study that followed diet soda drinkers for 9.5 yrs showed that the diet soda drinkers had a 5 times greater waist circumference than those who did not drink any soda or those who drank regular soda. However regular soda too should be avoided too due to the high sugar and calorie content.

- **Other Foods that are Ok to eat during the diet not listed on the original protocol:**
  - Mushrooms- 0 calories
  - Shirataki yam noodles- 0 calories (found in Asian Supermarkets or can be purchased off the internet). Shirataki noodles are 100% fiber and are not digested. They pass straight through the digestive tract and are eliminated in your bowel movement looking like noodles. So if you do eat these please do not be alarmed when you have a bowel movement. They can look like parasites/worms when they are eliminated in the bowel movement but this is totally normal and are just the noodles themselves.
  - Bragg's liquid amino acids- 0 calories. Tastes like a soy sauce substitute.
  - Note: Some people say coconut oil or MCT oil (Medium Chain Triglyceride) is ok to eat on the HCG diet due to the coconut oil being medium train triglycerides. Medium chain triglycerides are rapidly used/burned by the body for energy. However, in my personal experience of trying these, the oils made me stall out for about 2 days so I do not recommend them.
- **Pay attention to your total calories per day and your total carbohydrates. It is best to eat 50 or less grams of carbohydrates per day. This will put your body into a state of Ketosis which causes more rapid weight loss.**
- **It is ok to mix your vegetables during the HCG Diet. You will still lose weight and it makes it more enjoyable to have a variety of flavors to eat.**

The HCG Diet in a Nutshell

- **First 2 days: Loading Days:**
  - **Eat FATTY FOODS during the loading phase**. Contrary to the original Simeons HCG protocol, you do not have to eat until you are "stuffed." I had about 2 fatty food indulgences during my loading phase, as I did not want to gain weight and have to have a set back to lose it. Many people I see gain 2 or 3 lbs during the loading days and this is not necessary. You will give yourself **1 injection of HCG on each of these first 2 days**. Some examples of things to eat on this day would be: pizza, hamburgers, donuts, oils, avocados ice cream, olive oil etc.

- **21 Day Program: Next 19 days:**
- **30 Day Program: Next 28 days:**
- **40 Day Program: Next 38 days:**
  - Starting on Day 3 of the diet will be the 500 Calorie Diet. The daily injections are continued for the next 19 days combined with the 500 Calorie Diet.
  - *As soon as your statistically normal weight is reached, you may increase to 800-100 calories for the rest of the treatment.*

- **Last 72 Hours (aka. EXACTLY 3 days—must be exactly 72 hours from last HCG dose):**
  - **STOP the daily HCG injection** and continue to follow only the 500 calorie diet alone for 72 hours after the last HCG injection.

- **Maintenance Phase: Next 3 Weeks**
  - All foods are allowed except **no starch and sugar in any form** (careful with very sweet fruit).
  - Daily morning weighing is a must! If you will be traveling during this period then please remember to bring a scale with you on your trip.

- **Post-Maintenance Phase**
  - After 3 weeks, very gradually add starch in small quantities, always controlled by morning weighing.
  - Pay attention to any negative reactions that you experience when you add in a new food. This is a sign of a food allergy and if this occurs then avoidance of that food is a must.

The 500 Calorie HCG Diet

Breakfast	• Tea or coffee in any quantity <u>without sugar</u>. Stevia may be used. • Only one tablespoonful of milk allowed in 24 hours (Unsweetened almond milk works great for those who do not drink Cow's Milk, those who are lactose intolerant, for those with a food allergy to dairy) • MRM Whey Protein® sweetened with stevia 1 scoop in water (note: this contains Dairy) OR 3 egg whites with 1 cup of veggies (measured raw)
Lunch	1) 3.5 ounces (100 grams) of veal, beef (lean), chicken breast, fresh white fish, lobster, crab, or shrimp. All visible fat must be carefully removed before cooking, and the meat must be weighed raw. It must be boiled or grilled without additional fat. Salmon, eel, tuna, herring, dried or pickled fish are not allowed. *Limit beef to only 1-2 x per week 2) Vegetables to be chosen from the following (*it is ok to mix vegetables*): spinach, chard, chicory, beet-greens, green salad, tomatoes, celery, fennel, onions, red radishes, cucumbers, asparagus, cabbage, broccoli, cauliflower. (For meals 2 cups raw of veggies; If you are still hungry add another cup of raw veggies) 3) One Melba toast (plain) (OPTIONAL: Most people will find that they lose weight easier if they omit this). 4) An apple or 6 strawberries or one-half grapefruit or half cup of blueberries.
Dinner	The same four choices as lunch.

Note: If you are a tall woman 5'9'' or taller or a male 5'9'' tall or taller, you may increase your calories to 700 to 1000 calories per day. This can include increasing your ounces of protein at each meal or adding in an additional HCG meal (Lunch/Dinner) during the day.

In addition to staying at the proper calorie level each day, better weight loss results can be acquired by staying <u>at or below 50 grams of carbohydrates daily</u>. This will put your body into Ketosis resulting in more rapid weight loss.

Vegetarian HCG Options

Meat Substitutes:
- 1/2 cup of non-fat cottage cheese
- 1/2 cup of non-fat plain yogurt with no sugar added.
- Vegetarians who eat eggs can substitute 1 whole egg with the whites of three additional eggs served boiled or poached.
- There are some 'mostly' vegetarians who occasionally eat seafood. They can substitute shrimp, lobster, prawns, crawfish or crabmeat for the chicken or beef.
- Whey Protein, Pea Protein, or Hemp protein shake mixed in water. Make sure it is unsweetened or is sweetened with stevia.

Because of the starch content, vegetarians cannot eat the customary vegetable protein sources such as rice, beans, wheat or nuts.

If you can handle soy products, soymilk might be a safe alternative to cow's skim milk (or unsweetened almond milk), but you'd have to find a sugar-free/unsweetened version. It is also not recommended for men to eat soy due to the estrogenic effects of soy in the body.

Note: Because they don't eat the animal products called for in the original diet, strict vegetarians can expect their weight loss to be about half of that of the meat-eaters who follow this diet. This is what I have seen clinically in practice.

Spices Allowed During the 500 Calorie Diet

- The juice of one lemon daily is allowed for all purposes (3 Tablespoons of lemon juice per day)
- Vinegar (apple cider, white, red wine, but no balsamic or rice vinegar as balsamic and rice vinegars are too high in sugar content). (Due to being zero calories vinegar is unlimited for seasoning).
- Chicken broth, beef broth, and Vegetable broth- 1 cup per day is allowed for cooking purposes
- Salt, pepper, mustard powder, garlic, sweet basil, parsley, thyme, marjoram, etc., may be used for seasoning. Any dry seasoning that is free of sugar or fats/oils.
- NO OIL, BUTTER, MARGARINE, OR DRESSING IS ALLOWED.

Drinks/Beverages Allowed During the 500 Calorie Diet

- Tea, coffee, plain water (not from the tap—tap water contains chlorine which adversely affects the thyroid gland), or mineral water are the only drinks allowed, but they may be taken in any quantity and at all times. During the diet I liked putting flavored stevia such as Root Beer flavored Stevia into plain sparkling mineral water for a "Mock Soda." You can also use the flavored sparkling mineral waters as long as it is unsweetened and add regular stevia to it.

- You should drink half your body weight in ounces of water per day.
    - Example: If you weigh 200 lbs, then you drink 100 ounces of water per day.
    - Many patients are afraid to drink so much because they fear that this may make them retain more water. This is a wrong notion as the body is more inclined to store water when the intake falls below its normal requirements.

- The **fruit (or the melba toast- which I do not like people to eat the melba toast as it is empty carbohydrates)** may be eaten *between meals* instead of with lunch or dinner, but **NOT more than 4 items listed for lunch and dinner may be eaten at one meal.**

- There is no objection to breaking up the two meals. For instance having a melba toast and an apple for breakfast or before going to bed provided they are deducted from the regular meals. **The whole daily ration of two Melba toast or two fruits may not be eaten at the same time, nor can any item saved from the previous day be added on the following day.**
- The **100 grams of meat** must be scrupulously **weighed raw** *after all visible fat has been removed.* A food weighing/portioning scale must be used for measuring.

- Those patients who feel that even so little food is too much for them, can omit anything they wish.

A Stall. No Weight Loss for 3 Days in a Row. What do I do?

If you find yourself at the same weight for 3 days in a row there are 3 different options that you can do to jumpstart the weight loss.

How to break a stall in weight loss:

Option #1: An Apple Day

- This is a method used in the Reduction Phase to help break a stall in weight loss (aka. Plateau). **A stall would consist of no weight loss for 3 days in a row.**
- It consists of eating up to 6 apples of any variety and nothing more besides just enough pure water to satisfy an uncomfortable thirst throughout the day.
- According to Dr. Simeons, it is primarily psychological as the weight will continue to reduce without an Apple Day in good time, and the weight release after an Apple Day is primarily due to water loss. However, many people report a loss of about 2 lbs after an apple day.
- Drink the allowed beverages freely throughout the day especially water.

Option #2: A Protein Day

- Eat only the protein shake and/or meat all day without any vegetables, fruit, or Melba toast.
- Drink the allowed beverages freely throughout the day especially water.

Option #3: If #1 and/or #2 are not working

And if you find that Option 1 and/or 2 is not working it is then necessary to slightly increase your daily calories by 200 calories per day. Your body has probably gotten used to the 500 calories and has gone into starvation mode in which it will want to store fat and not release it. You would then increase either your protein portion sizes (i.e. eat 6 or 7 ounces of protein versus 3.5 ounces) or add an additional HCG meal to your daily diet menu.

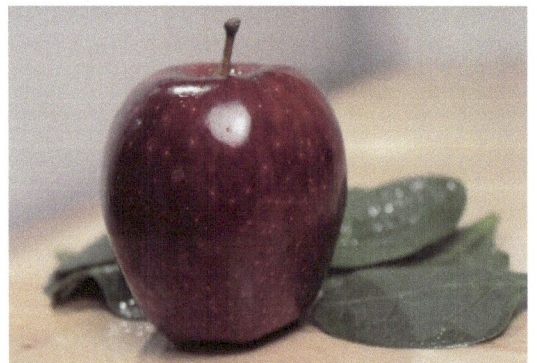

HCG Diet Safe Toiletries and Cosmetics

While on the HCG diet a strict rule is **no oils allowed**. If you check the ingredients in your personal hygiene products (i.e. shampoo, soap, shaving cream, etc.), there is most likely at least one type of oil in each product. You are cutting out all fat and oil while on the HCG diet, so if your skin comes into contact with any fats or oils, it will try and absorb as much as it can (as you are starving your body of fat so that it will use your own body fat for fats). Once you enter the Maintenance Phase of the diet then it is again acceptable to use personal hygiene and beauty products that contain oils/fats.

	What to Use while on the HCG Diet:
Cosmetics	Oil free cosmetics are allowed- Including any eye shadows, lipstick, and eyeliner.
Lip Balm	Carmex® or petroleum jelly.
Lotion	Most lotions or creams are not allowed as they often contain fat (i.e. Lanolin) and oil which will be absorbed into the body, which could cause weight gain or a weight loss stall while on HCG. If skin is dry and a moisturizer is needed then plain mineral oil can be used which has no nutritional value, or Aveeno® Unscented Oatmeal Lotion which contains dimethicone (a silicone/silica based oil).
Deodorant	Men's deodorant (Old Spice®, Axe®), crystal deodorant (wet crystal and apply), baking soda and/or cornstarch.
Toothpaste	Tom's of Maine® toothpaste, baking soda, or regular toothpaste can be used. I used regular toothpaste and it did not stall me out.
Soap	Zest, Ivory, Dial bar soaps. Avoid highly moisturizing soaps as they often contain oils.
Shampoo & Conditioner	Use any brand you want. Just make sure to rinse well and do not do any deep conditioning hair treatments while on the HCG diet.
Shaving Cream	Bar soap can be used to shave with

Proper Storage of your HCG

- Always keep your HCG refrigerated. If you will be traveling anywhere, always transport your HCG in a cooler with an ice pack or ice.
- Refrigerated HCG has a shelf life of 60 days.
- Accidently leaving your HCG outside of the fridge for more than 6 hours will make the mixture unstable and ineffective (i.e. it will lose it's potency). If this occurs it will be necessary to purchase a fresh batch of HCG from your doctor.

How to administer the HCG shots

- Clean the area with an alcohol swab in a circular motion, from center out.
- **Allowing the alcohol to completely air-dry will somewhat ease the discomfort of the shot.**
- Gently pinch the skin and insert the needle directly into it. Do not insert the needle completely into the skin. Inserting it ¾ of the way is perfect. These are subcutaneous injections, which means right under the skin.
- Pull back on the syringe slightly to check for blood in the syringe. If there is blood, simply reinsert the needle in another location.
- Inject the medication quickly or slowly- whichever is more comfortable for you.
- It is not abnormal to see a small amount of bleeding at the injection site. Direct pressure with a clean cotton ball or gauze will stop the bleeding and prevent bruising of the skin. **Slight** swelling, redness, burning, or itching is not uncommon and should subside shortly.
- **Helpful Measurements and Tips**
    - 1 ml = 1 cc
    - i.u. = International units

It is important that you use the recommended areas of the body for injection, as they will help ensure proper delivery of the medication to your system. **Subcutaneous injections should be administered to the lower abdomen, the upper and outer side quadrant of the thigh, the upper and outer quadrant of the buttock, or the upper outer arm. <u>Because repeated injections are required, and the skin may become red and tender, you should move the exact location about two inches from the previous injection site but still within the desired area and/or rotate injection sites.</u>**

<u>Also, it is important to know that injecting the HCG into a particular area on the body will not result in dissolution of fat in that area as HCG is not lipodissolve and is not a fat emulsifier.</u> Subcutaneous injection sites: Remember to rotate your injection sites daily!

How to take Oral HCG

If using oral HCG (prescription HCG, not homeopathic) then you must take the dose twice a day under the tongue. The medication does not last as long in the body when dosed sublingually versus an injection.

The following charts can be printed and can be used to track your weight loss by writing in your daily weight in each block/day.

Reduction Phase (21 Day Program)

1 Loading Day + HCG	2 Loading Day + HCG	3 500 cal + HCG WEIGH	4 500 cal + HCG WEIGH	5 500 cal + HCG WEIGH	6 500 cal + HCG WEIGH	7 500 cal + HCG WEIGH
8 500 cal + HCG WEIGH	9 500 cal + HCG WEIGH	10 500 cal + HCG WEIGH	11 500 cal + HCG WEIGH	12 500 cal + HCG WEIGH	13 500 cal + HCG WEIGH	14 500 cal + HCG WEIGH
15 500 cal + HCG WEIGH	16 500 cal + HCG WEIGH	17 500 cal + HCG WEIGH	18 500 cal + HCG WEIGH	19 500 cal + HCG WEIGH	20 500 cal + HCG WEIGH	21 500 cal + HCG WEIGH
1 500 cal only	2 500 cal only	3 500 cal only				

Maintenance Phase: 3 Weeks

1 Maintain	2 Maintain	3 Maintain	4 Maintain	5 Maintain	6 Maintain	7 Maintain
8 Maintain	9 Maintain	10 Maintain	11 Maintain	12 Maintain	13 Maintain	14 Maintain
15 Maintain	16 Maintain	17 Maintain	18 Maintain	19 Maintain	20 Maintain	21 Maintain

Reduction Phase (30 Day Program)

1 Loading Day + HCG	2 Loading Day + HCG	3 500 cal + HCG WEIGH	4 500 cal + HCG WEIGH	5 500 cal + HCG WEIGH	6 500 cal + HCG WEIGH	7 500 cal + HCG WEIGH
8 500 cal + HCG WEIGH	9 500 cal + HCG WEIGH	10 500 cal + HCG WEIGH	11 500 cal + HCG WEIGH	12 500 cal + HCG WEIGH	13 500 cal + HCG WEIGH	14 500 cal + HCG WEIGH
15 500 cal + HCG WEIGH	16 500 cal + HCG WEIGH	17 500 cal + HCG WEIGH	18 500 cal + HCG WEIGH	19 500 cal + HCG WEIGH	20 500 cal + HCG WEIGH	21 500 cal + HCG WEIGH
22 500 cal + HCG WEIGH	23 500 cal + HCG WEIGH	24 500 cal + HCG WEIGH	25 500 cal + HCG WEIGH	26 500 cal + HCG WEIGH	27 500 cal + HCG WEIGH	28 500 cal + HCG WEIGH
29 500 cal + HCG WEIGH	30 500 cal + HCG *Get your weight for this last injection day and record it.	1 500 cal only	2 500 cal only	3 500 cal only		

Maintenance Phase: 3 Weeks

1 Maintain	2 Maintain	3 Maintain	4 Maintain	5 Maintain	6 Maintain	7 Maintain
8 Maintain	9 Maintain	10 Maintain	11 Maintain	12 Maintain	13 Maintain	14 Maintain
15 Maintain	16 Maintain	17 Maintain	18 Maintain	19 Maintain	20 Maintain	21 Maintain

Reduction Phase (40 Day Program)

1 Loading Day + HCG	2 Loading Day + HCG	3 500 cal + HCG WEIGH	4 500 cal + HCG WEIGH	5 500 cal + HCG WEIGH	6 500 cal + HCG WEIGH	7 500 cal + HCG WEIGH
8 500 cal + HCG WEIGH	9 500 cal + HCG WEIGH	10 500 cal + HCG WEIGH	11 500 cal + HCG WEIGH	12 500 cal + HCG WEIGH	13 500 cal + HCG WEIGH	14 500 cal + HCG WEIGH
15 500 cal + HCG WEIGH	16 500 cal + HCG WEIGH	17 500 cal + HCG WEIGH	18 500 cal + HCG WEIGH	19 500 cal + HCG WEIGH	20 500 cal + HCG WEIGH	21 500 cal + HCG WEIGH
22 500 cal + HCG WEIGH	23 500 cal + HCG WEIGH	24 500 cal + HCG WEIGH	25 500 cal + HCG WEIGH	26 500 cal + HCG WEIGH	27 500 cal + HCG WEIGH	28 500 cal + HCG WEIGH
29 500 cal + HCG WEIGH	30 500 cal + HCG WEIGH	31 500 cal + HCG WEIGH	32 500 cal + HCG WEIGH	33 500 cal + HCG WEIGH	34 500 cal + HCG WEIGH	35 500 cal + HCG WEIGH
36 500 cal + HCG WEIGH	37 500 cal + HCG WEIGH	38 500 cal + HCG WEIGH	39 500 cal + HCG WEIGH	40 500 cal + HCG *Get your weight for this last injection day and record it.	1 500 cal only	2 500 cal only
3 500 cal only						

Maintenance Phase: 3 Weeks

1 Maintain	2 Maintain	3 Maintain	4 Maintain	5 Maintain	6 Maintain	7 Maintain
8 Maintain	9 Maintain	10 Maintain	11 Maintain	12 Maintain	13 Maintain	14 Maintain
15 Maintain	16 Maintain	17 Maintain	18 Maintain	19 Maintain	20 Maintain	21 Maintain

3 Week Maintenance Phase/Weight Stabilization Period

- The day that you give yourself your last injection, you count 72 hours (continuing on the 500 calorie diet for those 72 hours). Once the 72 hours is over, you begin the maintenance phase. **That weight that you were the morning of your last injection is the weight that you use as a basis for your maintenance phase.**

  NOTE: The time period to begin this phase is not 3 days after your last injection it is 72 hours! (For example, if you administer your last shot on Monday at 8 am, you will begin the maintenance phase on Thursday at 8 am.)

- First thing, when beginning the 3 week maintenance phase, **make sure to increase your calories to at least 1200 to 1500 calories/day.** Don't try to continue the diet after the HCG is out of your system. Make sure you are eating enough! Not eating enough can be counterproductive and lead to your body storing unwanted fat. **If you lose more than two pounds and did not want to lose any more weight, then add 100 more calories until you maintain your weight.**

- The Maintenance Phase is 21 days of eating regularly/eating whatever you want but **YOU MUST AVOID THE CARBOHYDRATES AND SUGAR. This is KEY to the success of this phase, which is weight stabilization at your new lower weight.**

- During this period patients must realize that carbohydrates (sugar, rice, bread, potatoes, pastries etc), are forbidden. If no carbohydrates whatsoever are eaten, fats can be indulged in somewhat more liberally and even small quantities of alcohol, such as a glass of wine with meals, does no harm. However *as soon as fats and starch are combined weight gain is for sure to happen*. The No Carb rule has to be observed very carefully during the first 3 weeks after the HCG Reduction Phase has ended otherwise weight gain/disappointments are almost inevitable.

- Drink enough water (half your body weight in ounces per day).

- **This is the period where your weight will stabilize.** Keep in mind, your weight will fluctuate the first week or two, which is normal. The weight will eventually stabilize. You will most likely continue to lose pounds during the Maintenance Phase.

- There are a few simple rules you must follow:
  - **YOU MUST WEIGH YOURSELF EVERYDAY (EVEN IF TRAVELING, TAKE A SCALE WITH YOU) after 1st emptying your bladder and before having breakfast.**
    - **You must remain within 2 pounds of your last injection weight (either above or below), and you CANNOT EAT SUGARS OR STARCHES! (wheat, barley, rye, oats, rice, pastries, pasta, corn, potatoes, carrots, beans, lentils)**
  - It is extremely important to eat enough protein on this phase. Many people eat at least 100 grams of true protein (about 400 grams weighed raw).
  - If you go **OVER the 2 pounds** (from your last injection weight), you must do a **STEAK DAY**: **This is used in Maintenance when one exceeds the 2 lbs difference from Last Dose Weight (LDW) to make a correction. It requires that one avoid all food until dinner when**

one is allowed to eat a large steak cooked in oil or butter and one apple. You drink water, tea, and coffee when you want and in whatever quantity you want during the day, but you do not eat anything until dinner.

Maintenance Phase: Low Carbohydrate Vegetables

This list is roughly arranged from lowest to highest carbohydrate counts, but all are non-starchy and generally low in carbohydrates. Exact carbohydrate count depends on serving size. Remember when counting carbohydrates in vegetables that the fiber is not counted, and can be subtracted from the total.

Low Carbohydrate Vegetables: EAT THESE!		Starchy (High Carbohydrate) Vegetables The **main veggies to be AVOIDED**
*Sprouts (bean, alfalfa, etc.) * Greens – lettuces, spinach, chard, etc. * Hearty Greens - collards, mustard greens, kale, etc. * Radicchio and endive count as greens * Herbs - parsley, cilantro, basil, rosemary, thyme, etc. * Bok Choy * Celery * Radishes * Sea Vegetables (Nori seaweed, etc) * Broccoli * Cauliflower *Cabbage (or sauerkraut) * Mushrooms * Jicama * Avocado * Cucumber (or pickles without added sugars)	*Peppers (all kinds) * Summer Squash (including zucchini) * Scallions or green onions * Asparagus * Bamboo Shoots * Leeks * Brussels Sprouts * Snow Peas (pods) * Green Beans and Wax Beans * Tomatoes * Eggplant * Artichoke Hearts * Fennel * Onions * Okra * Spaghetti Squash * Celery Root (Celeriac) * Carrots * Turnip (see Carbohydrate Counts of Root Vegetables) * Water Chestnuts * Pumpkin	* Beets * Carrots (depends on diet) * Corn * Parsnips * Peas * Plantains * Potatoes in all forms * Winter Squashes (particularly acorn and butternut)

Maintenance Phase: Low Sugar Fruit

In general, your best bet fruits are these, but do check carbohydrate counts. These are sort of arranged by sugar content, taking volume and weight, into account. This is not an exhaustive list. Good news: the fruits lowest in sugar are some of the highest in nutritional value, including antioxidants and other phytonutrients.

Fruits lowest in sugar:	Fruits fairly high in sugar:	Fruits to be AVOIDED in the maintenance phase:
* Rhubarb * Strawberries * Cranberries * Raspberries * Blackberries * Blueberries * Grapefruit * Melons * Apricots * Plums * Peaches * Pears * Guava * Cherries * Apples * Papaya	* Grapes * Tangerine * Oranges * Pineapple * Kiwi	* Bananas * Dried Fruit * Mango

Other Foods You Can Eat During the Maintenance Phase:

Eggs
Nuts
Nut butters
Oils
Avocados

Maintenance Phase:

Foods to Avoid:

Sugary foods: AVOID	Starchy foods: AVOID
Cookies	Cornstarch, corn, corn chips, popcorn, corn
cake	bread, corn meal
pie	white flour, wheat flour, any flour
candy	pasta
cupcakes	any bread or bread product: breadsticks,
frosting	bagels,
soft drinks	hamburger and hotdog buns, any breading on
corn syrup	fish, chicken or other protein, croutons,
Cool-aid	biscuits
processed food (i.e. Food that comes in a	crackers
box)	pretzels
energy drinks	tortillas, taco shells
fruit juice	oatmeal, Cream of Wheat
honey	rice, rice cakes
yogurt	polenta
donuts	peas
cookies	lentils
pudding	pita bread
maple syrup	yams
brownies	potatoes, potato chips
canned fruit in heavy syrup,	pancakes
ice cream	muffins
cool whip	nearly all root vegetables
boxed breakfast cereals	beans
breakfast bars	grains
granola	acorn squash, butternut squash
	cereals, cereal bars, protein bars, granola
	some nuts: acorn, coconut, chestnut

Be sure to read food labels, check to see if sugar is added into a product before you buy it. Nearly every product in a can or box contains sugar in one of its many names. The first five ingredients listed on an item is the majority of the product, so be sure that sugar is not in the top five.

Avoiding starch means avoid Most restaurants and fast food places add sugar to nearly every product, so be wary of eating out all the time. Other meats to watch out include deli meats, bacon, ham, prosciutto, sausage, and hotdogs.

Do not eat processed cheese (i.e. Velveeta), it contains unnecessary sugars and starches. Try not to eat processed anything for that matter.

Maintenance Phase:

Sample Daily Diet #1: Maintenance Phase	
Breakfast	2 Eggs (Hardboiled or scrambled with a little cheese)
	½ cup of low glycemic fruit or ½ of a grapefruit
	Tea or Coffee with stevia or unsweetened
Snack	1 ounce of raw unsalted almonds
Lunch	Chicken
	Vegetables
	Hard cheese or cottage cheese
Snack	Fruit (plum or apple)
Dinner	Baby field greens salad with feta cheese, avocado, tomato. Red wine vinegar and extra virgin olive oil for dressing.
	Unsweetened tea

Sample Daily Diet #2: Maintenance Phase	
Breakfast	Cottage cheese with strawberries
	Tea or coffee with stevia or unsweetened
Snack	Fruit (pick from the low sugar list)
Lunch	Mixed salad greens with chicken breast, walnuts, mandarin oranges, feta cheese and salad dressing *(make sure dressing does not contain corn syrup, honey, or fructose, sugar)*
Snack	1 ounce of Walnuts
Dinner	Salmon
	Vegetables
	Flavored Mineral Water (make sure unsweetened) with stevia

Done with Maintenance but you want to lose more weight? So you want to do another round of HCG. How long must you wait?

After completing the 3 weeks of maintenance, then one must wait another 3 weeks (6 weeks total) before starting another round of HCG. Failure to wait 6 weeks in between HCG rounds can possibly result in the HCG Diet losing effectiveness or immunity to the HCG can possibly occur.

Bonus: Sample HCG Diet Recipes:

Cajun Chicken Salad
3.5 ounces of boneless, skinless chicken breast 1 to 2 tsp of Cajun Seasoning 1 cup of chopped lettuce ½ chopped onion ½ sliced tomato Sea salt or Himalayan Salt to taste Black pepper Lemon Juice Rinse chicken breast and coat with the Cajun Seasoning. Grill or bake the chicken breast. Slice chicken and serve chicken over the lettuce, onion, and tomato. Sprinkle with salt, pepper, and lemon juice.

Hawaiian Chicken
3.5 ounces of chicken breast, cubed ½ cup of cabbage 1 clove of garlic minced 1 tsp of ginger 1 Tablespoon Braggs Liquid Aminos ¼ cup of water Fry chicken in pan with water, Braggs liquid Aminos, ginger, garlic, and cabbage.

Spicy Shrimp Gumbo
3.5 ounces shrimp 7 ounces of tomatoes 1 clove of Garlic Dash of Cayenne pepper (more if you like it spicier) Sea salt or Himalayan salt to taste Black pepper to taste 2 TBS Apple Cider Vinegar ¼ cup of water Place all ingredients into a saucepan. Simmer until the shrimp has turned white and the tomatoes have softened.

Other E-Books Coming Soon:
HCG Diet: The Doctor's Guide Cookbook. Healthy and delicious recipes to help you reach your weight loss goal.

Life After HCG Diet: The Doctor's Guide. How to eat healthy , make positive lifestyle changes, and keep the weight off after completing the HCG Diet.